LIGHT YOUR FIRE

The Ayurveda Diet

for
Weight Loss

ELAINE J. KELLER

TRUTH in 10 BOOKS

A Division of Brooklyn Indie Press
www.BrooklynIndiePress.com

I am, as always, utterly indebted to my parents and to the many teachings they have brought me.

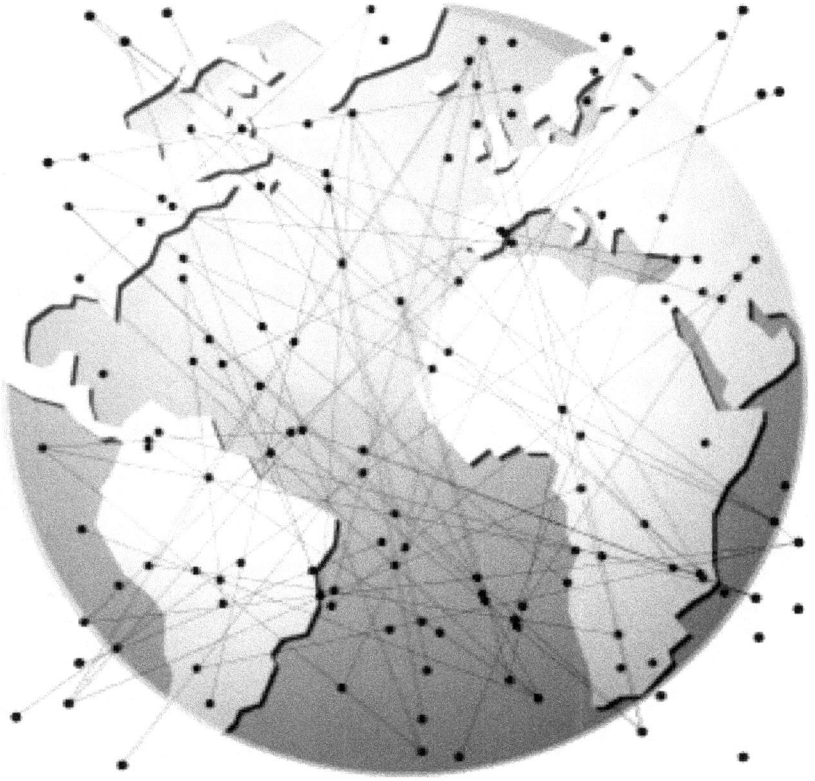

"... learn from one another, balance [Eastern] spirituality and [Western] material development."
—Paramahansa Yogananda, *Man's Eternal Quest*

TABLE OF CONTENTS

INTRODUCTION: Why Ayurveda?

Why The Western Lifestyle Fails

The Real Cause Of Weight Gain

Food As A Drug

Diet Products Create Obesity

Diets Don't Work

The Obesity Cycle Settles In

What's An Overweight Person To Do?

Why Ayurveda?

Why This Book?

Ayurveda Facts

The Ayurveda Diet

STEP 1: Create Ojas And Bring Vitality To Your Life

How To Produce Ojas

Forms Of Sugar

Pasteurization

To Create Ojas

STEP 2: Light Your Digestive Fire

Rest and Reset

Increasing Agni

STEP 3: Eliminate Amas

Identifying Ama

What Causes Ama?

How To Eliminate Ama

Ama Eliminating Diet

Easily Digested Foods & The Six Tastes

Ama Reducing Habits

STEP 4: Learn Your Dosha

Dosha Imbalance

Determining Your Dosha

Dosha Characteristics

STEP 5: Balance Your Dosha

How Imbalances Show Themselves

Balance Through Taste

Nourish Through Routine

Non-Kapha Weight Gain

STEP 6: Reduce Kapha
    Kapha Fitness
    Kapha Tips
    Kapha Reducing Plan

STEP 7: Cook With Weight-Reducing Herbs
    Spices That Aid Digestion
    To Control Blood Sugar
    Top Fat Busting Substances & Formulas

STEP 8: Combine Your Foods
    Fattening Food Combinations

STEP 9: Change Your Routine
    The Dosha Clock
    The Dosha Seasons

STEP 10: Institute Regular Detoxes
    Ama Detox
    DIY Panchakarma
    After Detoxing

STEP-BY-STEP: The Ayurveda Diet Guidelines

RESOURCES

    Dosha Quizzes

    Recipes

    Sources For Raw Honey, Raw Milk, Raw Butter, Non-GMO Organic Food

    Ama Detox Shopping List And Instructions

    Kapalabhati Instructions

    Guided Panchakarma

    Food Taste Lists

    Ayurvedic Herb Sources

REFERENCES

SHOPPING & COOKING LISTS

INTRODUCTION

WHY AYURVEDA?

Ayurveda is an ancient health system originating in India that embraces a whole and balanced existence. Its origin stems from the *Veda*, believed to be the word of *Brahma*, or the Hindu God. "*Veda*" means knowledge (science) or wisdom, and "*Ayur*" means life. Thus Ayurveda means "knowledge of life." Through Ayurveda we get to know our bodies, which are both run by, and are part of, the universal system of life.

What we eat, how we eat, and the manner in which we process the factors necessary for our existence, form the basis of this centuries-old science. In order to answer the question, "Why Ayurveda," it's necessary to launch into a quick description of our Western lifestyle.

Please forgive the following if it sounds harsh. We are at a critical juncture as human beings, where we are suffering needlessly from weight gain and obesity as well as a variety of dangerous illnesses. Once the problem is understood, the solution becomes simple and clear.

WHY THE WESTERN LIFESTYLE FAILS

Everything is fast these days.
Food...shopping...lifestyles...eating ... the time we take
for ourselves...physical activity... dealing with our
emotions...time spent with loved ones...

...and on, and on.

As a result obesity levels in the West are at an all-time
high, as are cancer rates, heart-disease, and a myriad of
life-threatening conditions.

THE REAL CAUSE OF WEIGHT GAIN

We are neglecting our physical and emotional well-
being. Microwaved dishes, processed meals,
consumable "food" products containing pesticides,
chemicals, additives, and synthetic substitutes are part
of a food supply that has been stripped of almost all
nutritional value, with its vital essence destroyed
through the processes of chemical adulteration,
synthetic reproduction and genetic modification.

Corporations have funded massive research endeavors
aimed at getting us to eat more by hijacking the
chemical processes in our brains, ratcheting up ever-
increasing dopamine levels in order create false
cravings and blocking the signals of being full. As a
result, we have become addicted to unnaturally sweet,
fatty, salty and "tasty" foods, and our taste buds no
longer recognize food that is good for us, and the
natural shut-off valve that tells us when to stop eating
has been eliminated.

This assault on our physical and mental bodies contributes to an ever-deepening spiral of weight gain, health problems and illness. Add to this the failure to exercise properly, lowered metabolisms, and lifestyles that deny us the time to nurture our spirituals elves, and we have retreated far from our intended natural state, which is one of health and well-being.

As those familiar with Eastern philosophy know, all things must be in balance for us to function as whole humans. Yet we Westerners are in a state of chronic imbalance.

Not just our physical selves are suffering, but our emotional selves as well. Failure to nurture our inner-being adds to physical disorders and weight gain. Additionally, when we neglect ourselves emotionally we eat more to comfort ourselves. When we fail to lose weight or to measure up to our idealized concept of ourselves we grow heavy with remorse, furthering the cycle of weight gain and illness.

FOOD AS A DRUG

Mike Adams, editor of *Natural News* reports:

"Bloomberg BusinessWeek exposes recent data that identifies junk food addiction as being as serious as drug addiction. High-fructose corn syrup (HFCS), monosodium glutamate (MSG), oils, refined salt, and other preservatives found in hydrogenated plentiful supply in our food does the same thing to a person's brain as cocaine does."

He goes on to say,

"A study conducted by researchers at the University of Texas in Austin (UT) and the Oregon Research Institute found that prolonged consumption of processed foods results in reduced activity in the section of the forebrain that registers reward. In other words, just like with illicit drugs, those addicted to processed food require ever-increasing amounts of it to get the same "high."

"You lose control. It's the hallmark of addiction," researcher Paul Kenny said.

In other words, Food = Drugs.

DIET PRODUCTS CREATE OBESITY

If this isn't enough, "diet" products cause us to gain weight.

A Purdue University study in the journal *Behavioral Neuroscience* reported that rats on diets containing the artificial sweetener saccharin gained more weight than rats given sugary food, casting doubt on the benefits of low-calorie sweeteners. Their research also shows that a group of test subjects fed artificial sweeteners subsequently consumed three times the calories of those given regular sugar. Diet soda, aspartame, etc. for weight loss, but in actual fact their advice causes the patients to crave calories and binge on unhealthy carbohydrates.

Fat-free products are not weight loss products at all and have an unnaturally high carbohydrate count, and increase our desire for more food. Obesity became epidemic in the West after the introduction of diet products into our food supply.

DIETS DON'T WORK

Yo-yo dieting is a common state for many of us, with the myriad of "newly discovered," "revolutionary," and "miraculous," diet plans failing to keep us slim and healthy in a lasting way. We grasp at the promise of new exercise regimes, equipment, drugs, and remedies in the hope that some new and miraculous product will rescue us from the fix we are in. Yet our efforts fail to provide more than a temporary solution, if any at all.

THE OBESITY CYCLE SETTLES IN

Partaking of diets with drastically lowered calories result in a lowered metabolism rate that leads to obesity. While they may deliver temporary weight loss, when the dieter returns to eating normally his slowed metabolism results in less food turning into more fat, launching us into the Obesity Cycle.

WHAT'S AN OVERWEIGHT PERSON TO DO?

A few facts to help put things in order:

o   Being overweight is a symptom, not an illness!

o   Obesity, yo-yo dieting, and weight gain are by-products of an out-of-balance body and lifestyle. The lack of nutrients available in our food these days causes us to eat more to absorb less.

o   If the underlying cause of the condition isn't addressed, the symptom of weight gain will continue, no matter how many diets you try.

This is because most diets don't address the weight gain at a core level.

If you put a Band-Aid on a cut finger it may heal, but it doesn't stop the action that caused the cut in the first place. If you continue slicing your finger, you will continue to bleed. Ibuprofen, acetaminophen, or aspirin relieve head pain, but they don't stop the cause. Dieting for the purpose of losing weight doesn't change the condition that created the weight gain to begin with.

To repeat, symptoms always return if you don't address the condition that caused them.

o   Lasting weight loss needs to be addressed holistically.

The Oxford Dictionary describes *Holism* as:

The theory that parts of a whole are in intimate interconnection that they cannot exist independently of the whole.

Man is more than blood, tissue and bone. We are more than flesh, water, brain matter, and emotions: we are synergistic, living organisms, whose parts contribute to a complex, thinking, spiritual, physical, *being*. When one part fails to work properly, the other parts are negatively affected. Ayurvedic philosophy states that we can not fix the resulting illness or condition without addressing the other facets of our beings as well.

In other words, all dietary regimes will be temporary or unhealthy until your whole self is addressed. This needs to be done in a holistic, synergistic way that deals with the *symptom* of being overweight.

We do this by balancing the hidden factors contributing to, or causing, our weight gain, whether it be:

- *toxic build up*
- *insulin resistance*
- *thyroid impairment*
- *sluggish metabolism*
- *failure to absorb nutrients*

...and more.

If your approach doesn't do this, YOUR DIET WILL FAIL

WHY AYURVEDA?

Ayurveda teaches us how to achieve perfection by creating harmony among all parts of our selves. For billions of people worldwide, it is embraced as an effective, comprehensive approach to building and maintaining health. Ayurveda's systematic method addresses bodily imbalance at its core level, creating a natural state of being that has no need of medicines, quick fixes, or ineffective dietary regimes.

Ayurveda does this by uncovering the body's imbalances and rectifying them with diet, herbs, exercise, and hands-on therapies. It is important to note that Ayurvedic herbal combinations are synergistic, and contain a variety of ingredients that work best when taken in conjunction with one another. A variety of herbs are available on the open market, and while they generally have no detrimental side effects, as always, seek qualified advice from a trained Ayurvedic doctor or health practitioner before taking new substances or embarking on this or any new diet program.

WHY THIS BOOK?

The science of Ayurveda is groundbreaking to Western thought in its comprehensive approach to obtaining optimum physical health in an efficient and balanced manner. By altering our habits in a small way we can critically effect the weight loss process.

We've taken the essential principles of this far-reaching science as they pertain to weight loss and have assimilated them into a pro-active and effective plan for achieving ideal body weight and maintaining it in a way that lasts.

AYURVEDA FACTS

1. What you eat, how you eat, and how you process the factors pertaining to your existence, form the basis of this centuries-old science.

2. The forces that comprise your body make-up are called *Doshas*. There are three of these: *Vata, Pitta,* and *Kapha*.

3. A person's unique blend of *Doshas* is known as *Prakriti*. An imbalance of one or more is called *Vikriti*.

4. *Vata* types are generally thin and underweight, and

suffer from excess anxiety.

5. *Pitta* imbalance can lead to digestive issues that cause weight gain or loss.

6. Excess *Kapha* leads to a slowed metabolism and extra weight.

7. A fiery *Agni*, or digestion, will increase metabolism and maximize weight loss no matter what your type.

8. Inefficient digestion creates *Ama*, the accumulation of toxic waste that turns to fat. *Ama* can be gotten rid of with a few simple lifestyle changes.

9. *Ojas* form the force of life that brings joy to your body and helps destroy *Ama*.

10. Cooking with herbs will speed up your metabolism, ignite your digestion, and eliminate toxins. Many herb combinations are unique to the Ayurveda and can be easily assimilated into your cooking routine.

THE AYURVEDA DIET

Before you begin: commit to yourself. Tell yourself you are going to completely and permanently lose weight by changing
the foods you take into your body and how you process them.

Take it one step at a time. Changing your lifestyle is a process.

The steps are explained in the chapters that follow.

Elaine J. Keller

Step 1:

Create *Ojas* and bring vitality to your life

Roughly translated, Ojas mean the "fluid of life."

When our life fluid is running freely and fully we are free from obesity and disease. *Ojas* is the vitality of life, creating a state of harmony as vital to our beings as water and sun.

Circulating *Ojas* vitalize tissues, sustain our hearts, clear our minds, nourish our life functions, and stabilize our emotions. *Ojas* also prevent a build-up of *Ama*, the accumulation of toxic waste that turns to fat. When Ojas are sapped or cut off, the body stagnates and is left unable to process fats and toxins.

Ojas are created from, among other things, completely digested and nourishing food.

HOW TO PRODUCE *OJAS*

Karta Purkh Singh Khalsa for *3HO Kundalini Yoga* describes Ojas as a "fine biological substance that comprises the most concentrated essence of nutrients and energy in the body." To fortify your precious *Ojas*, diet is key, Khalsa explains. "That diet needs to be a

highly nutritive program emphasizing whole grains like wheat and rice, seeds, nuts, milk products, and natural sugars, such as honey. " Cooked, moist foods (soups) add to this diet. Balance your diet to contain a broad range of all six of the Ayurvedic tastes: sweet, sour, salty, spicy, bitter, and astringent. "Generally, use food that is sweet, oily, cooling, light, and easily digestible, but cut back on dry or raw food," says Khalsa.
Make sure to include a organic raw (or cold-pressed) vegetable oil (almond, sesame) and ghee (recipe in Resources). Onion, garlic, ginger, eggplant, figs and dates all help build Ojas.
In our daily busy routine we are prone to eating processed or treated food without realizing that these are main causes of increased *Ama*. Essentially, food which is pure (or *sattvik*) and can be easily digested produce *Ojas*.

Let's examine the nutritional value of sugars and milks.

FORMS OF SUGAR

Honey

The practice of counting calories or the energy required to burn off a food item, is somewhat at odds with Ayurvedic thought which measures the value of food by its nutritive level in *addition* to its effect on bodily processes. The tendency of foods to help us shed or gain pounds is dictated by the way in which they synergize with other substances and interact with our body chemistry. Our bodies are working ecosystems either aided or hindered by the foods we ingest, with fat the byproduct of a "broken" system. In Ayurveda, the fattening quality of food is determined by the complete and synergistic effect it has on our bodies.

Our bodies interact in positive ways with whole foods and in toxic ways with those that are altered, dissected, refined or adulterated. This includes refined sugars, which are stripped of nutritive value as well as all of their healing properties.

Honey is a whole food, a substance which in its natural state produces a synergistic effect within our bodies, and which triggers our digestive fire when combined with warm water and lemon or cinnamon, for example.

Artificial sweeteners and refined sugars are considered toxins by our bodies, stripping us of vital metabolic energy and the resources needed to burn fat.

Raw honey's natural structure takes time to digest, causing its sugars to be released at a slower rate than other sugars. Honey is astringent and drying according to Ayurvedic teachings, which also stress that it is the only sweetener suitable for *Kapha* and effective in weight loss. There will be more about excess Kapha and its relation to weight gain, further on.

This does not mean to go crazy eating raw honey. Use in moderation, and in small amounts when trying to lose weight. Do not use processed sugars or sugar substitutes of any kind as these create toxins leading to fat.

It's worth noting that in a 2007 study in the *Journal of Food Science*, scientists found that rats fed with a honey-sweetened diet gained 23 percent less weight than those that consumed food sweetened with refined sugar over one year.

It is also important to know that heating honey in any

way, either by cooking, baking or adding it to hot beverages, creates toxic *Ama*. Only after a hot beverage has cooled to 104 degrees, can you add raw honey to it (above room temperature but far below boiling). Heating honey transforms it into indigestible matter that lodges in tissues. Make sure to eat your honey organic, raw, cold-processed, or straight from the honeycomb. Do not cook with it but add to tea after the liquid has cooled.

High Fructose Corn Syrup, Agave, Stevia, and Truvia

Refined sugars, high fructose corn syrup, and artificial sweeteners are *Ama* creating, and should be avoided at all cost.

The U.S. supply of agave, a cactus sugar which has recently gained popularity, has been found to be corrupted with high fructose corn syrup even though it is labeled "organic."

Stevia has long been used as a medicinal plant in South American cultures. Organically produced 100% stevia with no additives has not only been proven safe by these cultures, but also effective as a tool for reducing weight and for keeping glucose levels stable.

The brand name product "Truvia," is not pure stevia, but a derivative combined with additives creating an adulterated substance that is not proven to help lose weight and which, according to Ayurveda, will create toxins leading to fat.

PASTEURIZATION

Various studies have shown that heating honey, milk

and other vitally nutritious foods like almonds, kills their life force as well as amino acids, enzymes and minerals. This brings up the concept of pasteurization, which was created in the pre-penicillin era of filthy distillery dairies, when food products like milk spread deadly bacterial contagions.

Today's production standards and host of regulatory factors make pasteurization a largely unnecessary practice when it comes to domestic food products. The greater threat these days is eating foods devoid of nutritional value.

Thankfully, raw foods are available through select sources. It pays to be informed here and know that "raw" almonds, for instance, are pasteurized unless shipped from outside the U.S. (I have been eating almonds this way for years with no ill effects). Freeze upon delivery and thaw as needed in the fridge.

Raw Milk & Factory-Produced Cow's Milk

Raw milk, which is widely available in the Eastern world and certain American cultures, such as the Amish, consume on a daily basis without incident. The process of pasteurization (heating) used to slow down the microbial growth also destroys healthy bacteria or probiotics. While contrary to scientific and medical evidence that support pasteurization, it is considered immensely beneficial to drink raw milk. Try to locate sources of raw unpasteurized milk, or find milk that has been pasteurized with extremely low heat (see Resources). By all means look for organic, non-GMO milk without additives of any kind, even those deemed by manufacturers as "good for you."

Contrary to general popular belief, factory produced milk hinders the absorption of calcium and helps accelerate, if not create, a host of diseases. Ask yourself why the U.S. has a high consumption of dairy products and calcium, yet, it has one of the highest global rates of osteoporosis? Do not take anyone else's word as fact, including my own. Look into it yourself. Milk hurts asthmatics due to the production of harmful mucus in the body (*Ama*). According to *Naturasia*, UHT, or ultra-high processed milk contains minuscule particles that penetrate cell membranes which cause inflammation, leading to allergies, atherosclerosis and heart disease—and so on.

TO CREATE OJAS

Practice yoga
Practice *Prana Ama* breathing exercises
Get plenty of physical activity
Adopt a positive outlook
Eat a diet balanced with the six food tastes
Laugh often!
Follow your true path with respect to giving to others, not taking
Nourish yourself
Enjoy orgasms with the correct partner
Enjoy good digestion
Eat sweet foods like dates, natural seeds and nuts like almonds (soaked overnight and skin removed before eating on empty stomach)
Eat *Chyavanprash* (Ayurvedic jam)
Eat around people you enjoy
Meditate
Practice *Bhakti* yoga (devotion)
Learn controlled release of sexual energy
Cook with *Ghee*

When you are living a full life, free of guilt, toxins, remorse, fear, or regret; full of loving the correct partner, giving and receiving to and from others, nourishing your body and watching what you put into it, engaging in regular activities, eating, sleeping and exercising according to a general schedule, appreciating the beauty in all things, and creating with an open spirit-- the fluid of your life will be restored. This is the most vital and important step you can take in order to shed your excess weight.

Elaine J. Keller

Step 2:

Light Your Digestive Fire

We are what we digest.

Agni, or digestive fire , is a vital component of Ayurveda, and a fiery *Agni* is vital for weight loss. Highly functioning digestion enables us to absorb nutrients, and fires the metabolic processes that break down and transform food, creating heat to burn through toxins before they lodge in fat cells.

If our *Agni* is strong we are able to digest and assimilate food and perform well with high strength and vitality. Our body is less prone to diseases and does not accumulate toxins or fat. A strong *Agni* can help to diminish the aging process. Strong *Agni* digests our food at peak efficiency and helps us assimilate life's ups and downs. Weakened *Agni* cripples us physically and emotionally.

When our digestive fire is weak, toxic *Ama* lodges deep in our cells where it builds to produce excess fat and unhappiness, blocking the flow of life.

REST AND RESET

Ayurveda provides a tested method of igniting *Agni* and that has been proven to spur weight loss. It's called the *Agni* Reset.

Reset *Agni* weekly until losing your desired amount of weight. In general, reset twice a month for *Vata* and *Pitta* imbalance and once a week for *Kapha* imbalance.

Agni Reset

The process takes about two days and is easily done on weekends and prescribed as below. The process takes about two days. *Must Life* lays out the details:

Friday: Eat a normal breakfast and lunch. Eat a light, nourishing dinner. Before bed have three tablets of the laxative herb *senna*, followed by a glass of hot water. Go to bed early.

Saturday: In order to restart the digestive fire, you must first lower it. Therefore, on Saturday, only drinking is allowed. Apple or grape juice heated by adding hot water is easy on the stomach. Orange juice is too acidic. Have a glass at breakfast, one at lunch and another at dinner. Drink only three more during the day, otherwise drink water. The aim is to diminish your appetite with only minor calories to digest. Spend a quiet day reading. Be aware that toxins going into the mind can be as bad as toxins going in anywhere else.

Sunday: Eat a light breakfast of hot cereal with a cup of herbal tea. Licorice for *Vata*s, peppermint for *Pitta*s and *Kapha*s. Have a second helping of cereal if you need it. Do not eat again until noon when you should cook up a substantial, nourishing lunch. Have ginger tea with it to kindle the inner fire. At dinner, keep it light. Make sure you eat no less than three hours before bed. When you wake up, *Agni* will be blazing and ready to go!

Agni Reset Rules

Avoid alcohol, caffeine and cigarettes.
Eat at regular mealtimes and don't snack between meals.
Keep salt to a minimum and only have it with food.
Stick to recipes with foods appropriate to your *DOSHA* (see Resources)
If you get faint on day two, stir honey into your warm juice.
Only *Kapha*s can skip meals without upsetting their balance because their systems are relatively slow. Skipping meals compromises *Agni*.

INCREASING *AGNI*

Cook with herbs such as ginger, cayenne, and other spices that possess a warming, spicy quality (see Food Lists in *Resources*). These will help neutralize toxins especially if taken as teas, where they help kindle *Agni* and burn off toxins.

Fresh ginger root is the Ayurvedic "wonder root" that not only fires up digestion, but eliminates cramps, nausea, upset stomach, flatulence, vomiting and more. Drink a warm cup of ginger tea before meals, or suck on a piece of raw ginger sprinkled with lemon juice to fire digestion.

Fat is directly affected by the strength of your natural

digestion. If your *Agni* is strong and balanced then your fat metabolism will be normal or in a state of high performance. When *Agni* is functioning at a high rate, it breaks down food and assimilates it into the body while eliminating toxins and excess *Kapha*.

Step 3:

Eliminate *Ama*

Ama are toxins that turn to
fat in your body.

Inefficient digestion creates *Ama*, or the accumulation
of toxic waste that leads to weight gain. *Ama* clogs,
sticks, blocks, and clouds the body's channels and
creates the foundation for obesity and disease.

IDENTIFYING *AMA*

You probably have *Ama* in your body if you experience:

Atherosclerosis
Body aches and pains
Candida
Constipation or diarrhea
Foggy thinking
Gall stones, kidney stones
Gassiness, foul breath, stinky stools
High blood sugar levels
High liver enzymes
High triglycerides
Inability to focus
Lack of energy, fatigue
Lack of motivation
Late-onset diabetes

Low immunity, frequent colds, recurrent infections
Rheumatoid factor
Skin breakouts
Sluggish, bloated and dull feeling after meals
Depression

And particularly:
Weight gain

WHAT CAUSES *AMA*?

Caffeine, alcohol, cigarettes, drugs
Eating quickly and being distracted from eating
Watching television, working on the computer, or
reading while eating
Eating while emotionally upset
Eating food that is not pure, organic and fresh but old,
processed and packaged
Ice-cold drinks and cold-food meals
Irregular daily routine
Not making lunch the main meal
Not meditating regularly
Not moving your body regularly
Overeating
Poor diet
Stress

HOW TO ELIMINATE AMA

Herbs which are pungent and bitter in taste decrease
Ama, according to *Living Centre*. Some of these herbs
are:

Aloe Vera
Barberry
Black pepper

Cardamom
Cayenne pepper
Cinnamon
Fennel seeds
Ginger root
Guggulu - take this with Triphala.
Trikatu (black pepper, ginger, and *pippali* or Indian long pepper)
Triphala (*Amalaki, bibbitaki,* and *haritaki*)
Turmeric

Freely use these herbs when cooking.

AMA ELIMINATING DIET

The means to reduce Ama through diet is described by *Maharishi Yoga*. This simple diet consists of warm, freshly-cooked whole foods that are light, easy to digest, and are suitable for the person's body type and the season. It includes fresh, organic vegetables, sweet, juicy fruits, whole grains such as quinoa, rye, amaranth, barley, couscous, millet and rice, and easily digested proteins such as mung dhal or lentil soup (see *Resources* for recipes). Lassi is an excellent digestion-booster to drink after a meal because it contains acidophilus, a good bacteria that helps with digestion. (Note: Maharishi Yoga speaks of raw milk, which is widely available in India. Pasteurization destroys healthy bacteria as well as acidophilus. For this try to locate sources of raw unpasteurized milk, or find milk that has been pasteurized with extremely low heat (see *Resources*). By all means look for organic, non-GMO milk without additives of any kind, even those deemed by manufacturers as "good for you."

Cooked leafy greens such as chard and kale are especially good for improving elimination and detoxifying the body. Steam vegetables and grains with spices that are suitable for your body type of *Vata*, *Pitta* or *Kapha* such as *Churna* (see *Resources*). It is worth mentioning here the powerful detoxifying effect of Mung beans, which are believed to be highly nourishing and balance all three *Doshas*. They can be eaten in a soaked form as salad or soup. You can make your own detoxifying spice mixture by adding coriander, turmeric, and fennel. Turmeric is considered a primary tool to use in ridding *Ama* from the body, but take care to mix with other spices.

EASILY DIGESTED FOODS & THE SIX TASTES

The ancient texts on Ayurveda provide information on foods that are the most nourishing and most easily digestible, pinpointing, also, those most often found to be the source of illness. *Ayurveda* recommends the combination of tastes: sweet, pungent, salty, astringent, sour and bitter to produce full satisfaction to the body mind and soul. When you include all food tastes, it has a remarkable positive effect on your digestive power giving relief to you as a whole. A lack of all food tastes in the diet is not only depriving your taste buds but also your physical and emotional wellbeing.

Meats and grains which form main staple diet are considered to be sweet (or bland), spicy foods pungent and sour.

It is necessary to have a nourishing and easily digestible food in your daily diet to build healthy tissues to maintain various physiological functions at their best.

Following are lists for easily digestible foods with foods in bold are most nourishing and digestible (adopted from *Ayurveda Alchemy*)

Grains: Aged rice, millet, wheat, oats, couscous, rye, barley, amaranth

Cooked Vegetables: Squash, okra, radish, eggplant, sweet potato, bamboo shoots, bitter melon, spinach, onion, daikon radish, avocado, carrots, broccoli, parsnip, beets, asparagus, artichoke, bok choy, brussel spouts, burdock root, cabbage, cauliflower, green beans, leafy greens, peas, turnips, cauliflower, zucchini, kohlarabi, leeks

Fruits: Coconut, dates, grapes, mango, pomegranates, raisins, persimmons, apricot, banana, all berries, cherries, figs, grapefruit, kiwi, lemons, limes, oranges, papaya, plums, rhubarb prunes, pears, cranberries, strawberries

Legumes (soaked and well cooked): Mung beans, aduki beans, red lentils, chana dal, black-eyed peas, garbanzo, kidney beans, black beans, split peas, white beans, navy beans, pinto beans

Nuts & Seeds: Sesame seeds, almonds, charoli, pumpkin seeds, brazil nuts, cashews, coconut, hazelnut, macadamia nut, pecans, pistachio, walnuts, chia, flax seeds, sunflower seeds, hemp seeds, poppy seeds

Fresh Dairy: Raw cow's milk, ghee, butter, goat milk, home made buttermilk, unsalted cheese

Meat: Buffalo, bone broth, goat, rabbit, chicken, turkey, lamb

Occasional: beef, fish, seafood, duck, chicken eggs, duck eggs, pig

Sweeteners: Raw honey, jaggery, rock sugar, raw sugar cane, rapadura maple syrup, sucanat, agave, turbinado sugar

Oils: Sesame, ghee, unsalted butter, olive oil, peanut oil, coconut oil, flax oil (never heat), hemp oil, pumpkin seed oil

Spices: Most spices are beneficial; ginger, cumin, cardamom, fennel, coriander, cinnamon, saffron, turmeric, cilantro, dill, mint, neem leaves, black pepper, cayenne, chili, long pepper, cloves, garlic, horseradish, mustard seeds, nutmeg, onion, paprika, thyme, rosemary, sage, marjoram, hing.

When ill, do not take raw leafy greens and raw vegetables and avoid all fermented foods (sauerkraut, miso, kim chee, kombucha, soy sauce), Mushrooms, Sprouts, Tomatoes/Ketchup, Vinegar, Table Salt, Ice Cream, Cold Drinks, Smoothies, Fried & Fatty Foods, Cheese, Molasses, Frozen Food, Dried Meats & Vegetables, Leftovers, Sour Dough Bread, Processed and canned foods, Salted Butter.

Avoid cold food and drinks. Warm water drank throughout the day flushes out toxins. Speed up the process by making a tea with detoxifying spices.

AMA REDUCING HABITS

o Eat your main meal at noon, when the sun is strongest and the digestive fire reflects that strength. If you eat at different times each day, your digestion is thrown off.

o Don't eat at night, nor eat heavy foods such as meat or cheese, when the food will sit in your stomach. Eat at least three hours before bedtime so your food will be digested before you go to sleep.

o Eat at the same time every day so your body gets used to a routine, causing digestive juices to flow before the meal then working at top efficiently when you eat.

o Don't snack between meals unless you are hungry, and wait until food is digested before eating the next meal.

o Daily exercise stimulates digestion and helps cleanse toxins. It's also important to manage stress, and to have a job that you enjoy.

o Meditate each day to remove mental, emotional and physical stress.

Elaine J. Keller

Step 4:

Learn Your Dosha

The three Doshas are Vata, Pitta, and Kapha. Your constitution is a unique balance of each.

The core elements of fire, ether, air, earth and water comprise the *Doshas* that govern our bodies, interacting within our physical selves to form our *Pikrati*, or our uniquely individualized constitution. When in harmony, these forces combine to produce optimal health and body weight. When out of balance, illness and weight issues result.

Each *Dosha* is comprised of two of the elements:

- o *Vata* (air and ether)
- o *Pitta* (fire and water)
- o *Kapha* (water and earth)

Earth is the firmament which grounds and nourishes all living things.

Ether is the unlimited space which surrounds the earth and the planets. It is ever-present and all-encompassing, fueling interaction between the elements.

Air is the wind which carries *prana*, or life force, to all living things. The oxygen in air feeds our cells and maintains body functions.

Water in all its forms, whether steam, gas or liquid, is an essential nutrient for life.

Fire provides the body with heat and radiant energy that drives metabolic and chemical actions.

Prana or life force energy, powers the elements and governs all activity.

DOSHA IMBALANCE

Your *Dosha* was determined at the moment of your conception, when *Vata*, *Pitta* and *Kapha* uniquely joined to form you. From this moment onward your *Dosha* has been buffeted and soothed by elements within and without, creating strength in some areas and weaknesses in others. Factors affecting your *Dosha* include environmental conditions, what you eat, how you eat, and how you process the things you ingest—whether they be foods, environmental conditions, or emotions.

An imbalance in one or more Dosha is called *Vikriti*.

DETERMINING YOUR *DOSHA*

A number of *Dosha* tests are widely available. A quick search on the internet will produce dozens. But most of these contain ambiguous questions that are impossible to answer with accuracy.

The more comprehensive tests separate *Pikrati* from *Vikrati*, or your basic constitution type as well as areas of imbalance. Directions to these particular tests can be found in the *Resource* section.
Take a few and a pattern emerges. Are you mostly *Vata*, *Pitta*, or *Kapha*? Are you a blend of two primary *Doshas*? Are you a rare, balanced *Tri-Dosha*? Most people are a blend of two primary *Doshas* though we each possess some characteristics of each.

DOSHA CHARACTERISTICS

VATA: "The wind that moves things," or *Spacy Genius*

Unpredictable, enthusiastic, creative and spontaneous; a genius at expression and communication is *Vata* at its best. Able to think in highly intelligent, abstract ways, yet with short attention spans; too much *Vata* turns wind into a tornado. When *Vata* is in a weakened state, the wind can whistle through the trees of the brain as if no one is there. A *Vata* imbalance exhibits itself as nervousness, hypersensitivity, difficulty finishing tasks, and giving up too easily. Physically it manifests in low body weight, gas, constipation, sensitivity to cold, jumpy behavior, insomnia, anorexia, and forgetfulness.

To balance excess *Vata*: establish yourself in a routine, eat warming foods and focus on one thing at a time. Use a timer and allot specific amounts of time for each task. Be *present* in interactions with others.

PITTA: "The transformer," or *Assertive Entrepreneur*

Orderly, focused, intelligent, and articulate, *Pitta*'s fiery passion ignites desire in others. At best *Pitta* is a joyful and courageous leader. At worst, *Pitta* flares into a raging firestorm becoming combustible, pushy, controlling, and bitter.

Excess *Pitta* energy consumes others in its self-created hellfire. Too stressed to eat regular meals, unbalanced *Pitta* soars from overwork and manifests in impatience, criticism, intolerance, and an overbearing nature. Physical imbalances run hot with infections, acid reflux, heartburn, ulcers, ravenous hunger, out-of-control cravings and emotional overeating.

To balance excess *Pitta*: go on a mountain hike or canoe down a river. Stay out of the sun. Don't eat when you're stressed or angry. Cut out the competitiveness and stop overworking.

KAPHA: "The glue that binds," or *Earth Mother*

Easy, affectionate, and non-judgmental, *Kapha*'s earth/water energy is a calm and enduring stream, and does not burn itself out like Pita, or run cold like *Vata*. Loving, compassionate, and forgiving when in its balanced state, *Kapha* out of control hardens into plodding, jealousy, implacability, or outright laziness. Stability turns into inertia, with obesity a common result as well as physical ailments like sinus congestion, colds and allergies.

To balance excess *Kapha*: engage in daily physical activities. Mow the grass, jog to the grocery store, and park in the farthest spot from your destination. Take the stairs and avoid the escalator. Break a sweat, and never idly watch TV. When stuck, break routine.

KEEP YOURSELF IN BALANCE

Factors that create imbalance are the foods we eat, the way we eat, our lifestyle, our emotional levels, the manner and extent of our physical exertion, physical and mental trauma, and so on. Common sense plays a big part in bringing ourselves into balance.

PITTA is governed by fire, so engage in foods and activities that are cooling.

Food tastes to embrace: Astringent, bitter, sweet

Food tastes to avoid: Pungent, sour, salty

Avoid: Talking about yourself and skipping meals.

VATA is governed by wind and cold, so to balance *Vata* engage in activities and foods that are warming.

Food tastes to embrace: Sweet, sour, salty

Food tastes to avoid: Pungent, bitter, astringent

Avoid: anything cold, like winter hiking expeditions and ice cream.

KAPHA is governed by earth and water, so engage in activities and foods that are stimulating and drying.

Food tastes to embrace: Pungent, bitter, & astringent

Food tastes to avoid: Sour, salty, sweet

Avoid: Swampy jungles, soap operas, and M&M's.

Season, weather and environmental conditions affect our state of balance. Winter or cold creates excess *Pitta*. Blustery wind creates excess *Vata*. *Kapha*s are slowed down by damp weather. As you become attuned to your nature you will start to feel imbalances naturally. At these times take extra care to eat according to your *Dosha* and engage in *Agni Reset* and *Panchakarma* (described in the sections that follow).

For a large part, weight gain is excess *Kapha* in an out-of-balance constitution. Dietary and lifestyle changes to bring *Kapha* under control will be described further along in the book.

Step 5:

Balance Your *Dosha*

Following some dietary guidelines will help balance Vata, Pitta, & Kapha

When we don't eat according to our *DOSHA* we perpetuate imbalance. *Pittas* who eat spicy foods over a prolonged period develop chronic heartburn. Vatas eating astringent food develop gas and constipation and have trouble sleeping through the night. *Kapha* puts on weight.

HOW IMBALANCES SHOW THEMSELVES

Vata: associated with air and motion, including circulation, breathing, blinking, and heartbeats, when *Vata* is out of balance nervous problems such as hyperactivity and sleeplessness, as well as lower back pains and headaches result.

Pitta: related to metabolism, body heat, digestion and absorption of nutrients. *Pitta* imbalance is often stress-related and shows up in conditions like ulcers, gastritis, and hypertension.

Kapha: controls growth in the body and supplies water to body parts, moisturizing the skin, and maintaining the immune system. *Kapha* imbalance results in obesity, fatigue, bronchitis, and sinus problems.

BALANCE THROUGH TASTE

The taste of a food helps determine its ability to balance each *DOSHA*, whether it is bitter, pungent, astringent, salty, sour, or sweet.

Dr. James Brooks, author of *Ayurvedic Secrets to Longevity and Total Health* notes that the average fast food diet of hamburger, French fries, coke and ketchup has only three of these tastes: sweet, salty, and sour. These are *Vata* pacifying. *Vata* imbalance is very common in Western society due to a fast paced lifestyle and the over-reliance on fast food.

Dr. Kulreet Chaudhary helps define the balancing nature of foods by their taste:

BITTER: lessens *Kapha* and *Pitta*, increases *Vata*

Includes vegetables such as chicory and bitter gourd; green leafy vegetables such as spinach, green cabbage, and brussel sprouts; fruits such as olives, grapefruit, and cocoa; spices such as fenugreek and turmeric

PUNGENT: lessens *Kapha*, increases *Pitta* and *Vata*

Spices such as cardamom, chili, mustard seeds, cumin, black pepper, ginger, cloves, garlic; mild spices such as turmeric, anise, cinnamon, and fresh herbs such as oregano, thyme, mint; raw vegetables like onion, cauliflower and radish

ASTRINGENT: lessens *Pitta* and *Kapha*, increases *Vata*

Turmeric, honey, walnuts, and hazelnuts; pulses such as lentils, peas, beans; green leafy vegetables like lettuce, sprouts, and raw vegetables; fruits like berries, pomegranate, and apple

SALTY: lessens *Vata*, increases *Kapha* and *Pitta*

Any kind of salt or food which is salted.

SOUR: lessens *Vata*, increases *Kapha* and *Pitta*

Sour fruits such as lemon and lime, passion fruit, sour cherries, and tamarind; sour milk products such as yogurt, cheese, whey, and sour cream; fermented substances (other than cultured milk products) such as wine, vinegar, soy sauce, or sour cabbage; carbonated beverages (including soft drinks or beer)

SWEET: lessens *Pitta* and *Vata*, increases *Kapha*

Most grains such as wheat, rice, barley, and corn; pulses (legumes), such as beans, lentils, and peas; milk and sweet milk products such as butter, cream and ghee; sweet fruits (especially dried) such as figs, grapes, pear, dates, coconut, and mango; cooked vegetables such as sweet potato, carrot, beet, potato, and cauliflower; sugar in any form such as raw, refined sugar, brown sugar, molasses, and sugar cane

NOURISH THROUGH ROUTINE

Diet as well as routine should be used to balance your constitution. Nadya Andreeva of *Mind Body Green* stresses
that Vata types should include cooked, warm foods, stay away from icy drinks, and add warming spices like cinnamon, cloves, and ginger to their food. The following tips contain her general guidelines for each *Dosha*.

VATA: Stay warm

Be regular in your routine; eat and go to bed at a consistent hour, get enough sleep, and choose foods that are warm, cooked and nourishing; berries, rice, fruits, nuts and dairy products are good choices for *Vata* types.
Exercise moderately. A more meditative yoga, Tai chi, walking, and swimming are recommended. Avoid strenuous activities.

PITTA: Stay Cool

Avoid overexposure to direct sunlight
Avoid fried and spicy foods
Avoid alcohol and tobacco, don't overwork or become overheated.
Be regular in your routine; eat and go to bed at a consistent hour, get enough sleep
Choose fresh vegetables and fruits that are sweet and watery like mangoes, cucumbers, cherries, avocado and water melon
Eat lots of salads with dark greens such as kale, arugula, and swiss chard
Avoid conflicts

KAPHA: Get Moving

Get out of the house and seek new experiences
Be receptive to useful change; be intentional in
implementing life-enhancing actions Choose foods that
are light, warm, and spicy
Tea with ginger and lemon as a great pick-me-up
Avoid heavy oily and processed sugars
Use lots of spices such as black pepper, ginger, cumin,
chili and lots of bitter dark greens.

NON-*KAPHA* WEIGHT GAIN

While often the culprit, Kapha is not always the only
imbalance to cause weight gain.

Claudia Ward, L.Ac, of BEYOND ACUPUNCTURE, addresses
the issue. "Those with a Vata imbalance gain weight
when anxious, burdened or exhausted from too much
work. Vata imbalance can result in food addiction
because they need regular meals that are nourishing,
and made with warming spices and healthy fats. Protein
shakes, green drinks, raw salads and coconut oil are
counterindicated for Vata imbalance," she states.
"While healthy for some, coconut oil is cold in nature
and clogs the channels. Crackers, chips and rice cakes
should also be avoided."

Pitta types, she says, need regular meals that are lightly
cooked with plenty of dark green bitter vegetables,
summer squashes, asparagus, green beans and mild
spices such as fennel or coriander. Juicy pears are a
good healthy treat for Pitta's sweet tooth.

Kapha individuals need to get moving to counteract

their sedentary tendencies. Warming spices and foods are recommended, Ward says, as are bitter leafy greens and fresh herbs. Cold drinks, coconut oil and raw salads should be avoided.

Step 6:

Reduce *Kapha*

Kapha imbalance =fat.

For a large part, weight gain is excess *Kapha* in an out-of-balance constitution. *Kapha* is caused by slow metabolism which results in the body's inability to digest or break down food into energy, resulting in accumulation of toxins or excess fat. *Kapha* weight gain is also accompanied by retention of water and aided by excess intake of salt.

Dietary and lifestyle changes including regular exercise regimes, are necessary to bring *Kapha* under control. Here are the words you may not want to hear: for *Kapha*, exercise is the key.

The more you exercise the better it is. *Kapha*'s slowed-system is reversed through exercise. There's nothing new here; everyone knows you must exercise to reduce fat. Yet the quality of exercise along with right diet is important. *Kapha* exercise should be vigorous but never extreme.

KAPHA FITNESS

Kapha needs to exercise every single day, no matter what. Focus on vigorous movement and practice yoga, walking, running and swimming. Use a mini-trampoline, weighted hula hoop, or dance to energizing music.

The *Chopra Center* states that any kind of aerobic activity that works up a good sweat is powerful for clearing Kapha congestion and sluggishness.

Any vigorous calorie-burning activities will reduce *Kapha* immensely and enhance flexibility and mobility. In many Ayurvedic centers located in India, energy intensive sports like *kushti* (wrestling) and *kabbadi* sports are played in order to keep fit.

Yoga is ah excellent activity to revitalize overall health. *Ayurvedic Health Center* states that in order to alleviate Kapha excess in the body, "one must consider using opposites." So, the yoga practice should be conducted in a warm, dry environment with nice bright, energetic colors and music. The practice should be fast-paced, using a *vinyasa* flow (movement synchronized to the breath) that is dynamic and meant to raise heat in the body. The *drishti* (gaze) should be upward whenever possible and the palms facing up, fingers spread and strong. The focus should be on expanding the 4th and 5th *chakras* (heart and solar plexus), so backbends are great. Inversions like these help increase circulation in the head and chest. Engaging the larger muscles (e.g. quadriceps), helps increase heat quickly in the body, thus the Warrior poses are great additions. The student should focus on bringing intensity and strength to the poses, engaging the muscles firmly. The keys are dynamic movement, upward energy, and heat.

The ideal breathing exercise for *Kapha* balancing is *Kapalabhati* (see Resources). It clears the lungs, increases heat in the body, tones the abdomen, burns fat, and creates a sense of lightness, and combats lethargy.

KAPHA TIPS

Don't drink cold liquids after exercise. This will hinder the cells from burning more calories and from increasing fire.

No napping during the day. Reducing *Kapha* demands an active lifestyle.

Mustard oil or strong massage with light oils such as linseed aids weight loss and eliminates toxins.

KAPHA REDUCING PLAN

Kapha-aggravating foods as generally those that are sweet, heavy , salty, oily, sour and greasy. Utilize herbs to light the fires of digestion and freely incorporate green leafy vegetables into your diet. Fruits such as berries, grapefruits, pears, papayas and apples are considered stimulating to *Kapha* sluggishness. Others, such as pineapple or watermelon are too sweet and add weight. Dairy creates mucous and slows *Kapha* down, and should be eliminated. Low-fat yogurt or ghee is okay in moderation. Red meat should be replaced with chicken, turkey, or freshwater fish like catfish or trout. Tilapia is considered a freshwater fish, but has become contaminated by today's food producing methods. Eliminate sugar, wheat, nuts, salty, greasy and refined foods. Drink water, and lot's of it. Cook with warming, pungent spices such as black pepper, chili, cumin, ginger and cayenne.

You are probably reading this list and asking, "well doesn't this apply to everyone? It sounds like a dietary list for healthy living to me." The fact is that Westerners in general are suffering from excess *Kapha*.

So what does a *Kapha* reducing diet look like?

Beans are great for *Kapha*. Start with the mung bean soup for three to five days. Add in veggies, poultry or freshwater fish sautéed lightly with ghee, or for quicker reduction, steamed.
Freely cook with ginger, turmeric, cayenne, black pepper, cumin, fennel, cinnamon, and coriander. Eat at regular times. More will be discussed in the following chapters, but staying on a schedule is very important for reducing *Kapha*. Avoid drinks that are cold, and exercise every day.

Step 7:

Cook with weight-reducing herbs

*Learn the herb combinations
that banish fat.*

Ayurveda promotes herbs and spices as one and the
same. Whether incorporated into your meals or taken
on their own, their assistance is integral to losing
weight and keeping it off. Many herbs make foods more
digestible by "predigesting" the ingredients during
cooking, like, for instance, long pepper, black pepper,
cayenne, cardamom and licorice.

Fennel is a multifunctional herb used as a fat
metabolizer, appetite suppressant and to prevent gas.
In Indian restaurants a plate of fennel seeds is generally
available at the counter. The idea is to chew on a
teaspoon of seeds, spit out the pulp and swallow the
juice.

Asafetida (*hing*) is used in cooking or in the preparation
hingavashtak, where it is mixed with other herbs to
promote assimilation of nutrients. It is used to aid
digestion. Its drying, warming, and stimulating actions
awaken *Agni* and tones the digestive system.

Some Other Great Herbs and Spices:

Cinnamon soothes the stomach and is known to lower LDL, the "bad cholesterol" and increase HDL, or the "good cholesterol." It also helps lower blood sugar levels and improves insulin sensitivity.

Cumin is a powerful digestive, flushes out toxins, improves absorption and digestion, and helps assimilate nutrients in the body. It also supplies a thermogenic or fat-burning effect.

Ginger is highly effective in stimulating digestion and facilitating transport of nutrients to tissues while clearing blockages from body channels.

Gymnema sylvestre destroys the taste and craving for sugar, and regulates blood sugar levels.

Trikatu improves metabolism and destroys *Kapha*.

Triphala is known for its cleansing action and supports weight loss.

Triphala Guggulu aids fat metabolism and detoxification. According to various books of Ayurveda, *Triphala Guggulu* is a wonder herb combination, which cures almost all the ailments that are present on the earth. The intense bitterness of *neem* (in combination) cleanses blood and refreshes palates.

Triphala Guggulu balances *Vata* (Air), *Pitta* (Metabolic Fire), and *Kapha* (Water) in the body.

Turmeric controls blood sugar levels, promotes thermogenesis and enhances detoxification of the liver. Liver health is vital for regulating sugar and fat metabolism.

Black pepper improves circulation and digestion, while its heating effect boosts metabolism for weight loss. Piperine, an alkaloid contained in black pepper, suppresses accumulation of body fat, helps detox waste and enhances bioavailability of nutrients when consumed with other herbs and foods.

SPICES THAT AID DIGESTION

Ajmoda (celery seed, leaf, root, stalk)
Asafetida
Cayenne
Chyavanprash (jam)
Coriander
Cumin (jeera)
Fennel
Ginger
Hingwastaka
Kalijeera (bitter cumin)
Pippali
Trikatu (ginger, long pepper, and black pepper)
Trikulu (clove, cardoman, cinnamon)
Turmeric

TO CONTROL BLOOD SUGAR

Ashwagandha
Neem
Turmeric

SUPPORTS ELIMINATION

Fresh curry leaves
Chyavanprash

TOP FAT BUSTING SUBSTANCES & FORMULAS

Shilajit: "Toxic Destroyer"

Shilajit is Ayurveda's great detoxifier. Its prime
ingredient, fulvic acid, neutralizes free radicals and
detoxifies on a grand scale. *Shilajit* is described as
containing over 85 minerals and trace elements while
its high concentration of fulvic acid helps the body
absorb these minerals at a cellular level. It's best to look
for high quality, authentic, pure Himalayan *Shilajit*.
Like other herbs it has a synergistic effect when used in
conjunction with others, and it's best not to isolate
compounds and take it alone such as pure fulvic acid.
Take a pea size amount once or twice a day, under the
tongue or dissolved in warm water.

Trikatu: "Fiery Avenger"

Trikatu consists of three herbs: black pepper, ginger
and pippli. This synergistic warming formula awakens
Agni and destroys *Ama* while enhancing metabolic
activity and absorption of nutrients.

The information given in the Ayurveda writings prescribes as follows:

1/2 to 1 teaspoon one hour before each meal. It's also effective along with or after a meal. As *Trikatu* has a pungent taste, it can be mixed with honey to make a thick paste and consumed that way.

Foods which are inferior in value and are eaten in untimely manner give rise to the upper GI health problems as well as increased appetite and cravings. *Trikatu* helps to maintain the healthy digestive system and removes the toxins from the body. It was shown to reduce LDL and triglycerides levels in rabbits fed high-fat diets. It also increased cardio protective HDS levels. *Trikatu* is an especially helpful combination of herbs for preventing obesity.

Triphala: "Slayer of Stagnant Bowels"

Possibly the most well-known Ayurvedic formula is *Triphala*, or "three fruits." These are *amla*, *bibhitaki*, and *haritaki*. A general detoxifier and antioxidant, Triphala has a light laxative effect.

Hingavashtak: "The Planter"

Promoting deep assimilation of nutrients, especially in the small intestine, *hingavashtak* helps maintain friendly flora in the lower intestines while promoting destruction of parasites. The aromatic spices decrease *Vata*-type afflictions such as gas and bloating while supporting *Agni*.

Guggul/Triphala Guggulu: "Fat Banisher"

Guggul regulates metabolism and suppresses appetite. Mixed with triphala, guggulu helps release excess Kapha from the system, minimizes Ama and supports Agni. According to *Baba Rambev*, "Triphala Guggul combines the detoxifying and rejuvenating actions of triphala with the deeply penetrating and cleansing actions of Guggul. Triphala Guggul decongests the channels of the body and scrapes away toxins held within the tissues."

Step 8:

Combine Your Foods

*Avoid eating certain foods with one another
to increase weight loss.*

The manner in which we combine certain foods, and the amounts in which we eat them determines how well we digest their nutrients and unleash their beneficial qualities.

Food combinations are of great importance to stimulating *Agni* and reducing *Ama.* Vasant Lad of the *Ayurvedic Institute*, explains that according to Ayurveda, "every food has its own taste (rasa), a heating or cooling energy (virya) and a post-digestive effect (vipaka). Some also possess *prabhava*, an unexplained effect. So while it is true that an individual's *Agni* largely determines how well or poorly food is digested, food combinations are also of great importance. When two or more foods having different taste, energy and post-digestive effect are combined, Agni can become overloaded, inhibiting the enzyme system and resulting in the production of toxins. Yet these same foods, if eaten separately, might well stimulate Agni, be digested more quickly and even help to burn Ama."

Fruit should always be consumed by itself, Lad instructs in his paper, *Food Combining*, as they create an "indigestible wine" in the stomach when eaten with other foods.

According to Lad there are some incompatible foods not worth combining:

Beans with... *fruit, cheese, eggs, fish, milk, meat, yogurt*
Eggs with... *fruit, especially melons, beans, cheese, fish, khitchari, MILK (especially), meat, yogurt*
Fruit, as a rule, without *any other food.*
Grains with...*fruit (especially acidic or sour taste), tapioca*
Honey with... *ghee*
Hot drinks with... *mangos, cheese, fish, meat, starch, yogurt*
Lemon with... *cucumbers, milk, tomatoes, yogurt*
Melons *should be eaten alone.*
Milk with *BANANAS (especially), cherries, melons, sour fruits; bread containing yeast, fish, khitchari, meat, yogurt*
Nightshades e.g., potato, tomato... with *melon, cucumber, dairy products*
Radishes with... *bananas, raisins; milk*
Tapioca with... *fruit, especially banana and mango; beans, raisins, jaggery*
Yogurt with... *fruit, cheese, eggs, fish, hot drinks, meat,*
Milk with... *nightshades*

Specific common food incompatibilities are listed below.

INCOMPATIBLE FOOD COMBINATIONS

Milk Is Incompatible With:

o Bananas
o Fish
o Meat
o Melons
o Curd
o Sour Fruits
o Khitchari
o Bread containing yeast
o Cherries

Melons Are Incompatible With:

o Grains
o Starch
o Fried foods
o Cheese

Starches Are Incompatible With:

o Eggs
o Milk
o Bananas
o Dates

Honey Is Incompatible With:

o Ghee (in equal proportions)
o Heating or cooking with.

Radishes Are Incompatible With:

o Milk

o Bananas
o Raisins

Nightshades, (Potato, Tomato, Chilies) Are Incompatible With:

o Yogurt
o Milk
o Melon
o Cucumber

Yogurt Is Incompatible With:

o Milk
o Sour Fruits
o Melons
o Hot drinks
o Meat
o Fish
o Mangoes
o Starch

Eggs Are Incompatible With:

o Milk
o Meat
o Yogurt
o Melons
o Cheese
o Fish
o Bananas

Mangos Are Incompatible With:

o Yogurt
o Cheese

o   Cucumbers

Corn Is Incompatible With:

o   Dates
o   Raisins
o   Bananas

Lemon Is Incompatible With:

o   Yogurt
o   Milk
o   Cucumbers
o   Tomatoes

Elaine J. Keller

Step 9:

Change Your Routine

A daily routine with regard to when you eat, sleep, work, and exercise is essential for lasting change.

THE DOSHA CLOCK

Just as the Dosha govern our constitutions, these energies govern the hours of the day. Obviously it is impossible to embrace these changes all at once. Incorporating the routine gradually, as you can, will help further a lasting change.

Kapha (6 – 10 a.m., 6 – 10 p.m.) Stable Energy, "Routine"

A time when our deepest habits are established. Use this time to exercise and meditate, especially in the morning and develop an enduring habit. Morning *Kapha* hours are ideal, with evening hours being a useful alternative.

Pitta (10 a.m. – 2 p.m., 10 p.m. – 2 a.m.) Concentration

and Focus, "Second Wind"

Pitta heat governs digestion and appetite so it is wise to eat the biggest meal of the day at lunch. As *Pitta* energy is to blame for compulsive eating and dreaded midnight snacking, it's best to be asleep by 10 p.m.

Vata (2 – 6 p.m., 2 – 6 a.m.) Spontaneity and Imagination, "Creative Time"

Vata's windy unpredictability makes it difficult to establish routine. Use these hours to learn, create, study, or work on projects.

Sleeping and Waking

If at all possible, go to sleep by 10 p.m., because during the *Pitta* time of night of 10 p.m. –2 a.m. your digestion has a chance to cleanse and rejuvenate itself. If you stay up you'll undoubtedly get hungry again.

Waking before 6 a.m. is recommended. Sleeping into morning *Kapha* time of 6–10 a.m. clogs the channels of your body and creates *Ama*.

THE DOSHA SEASONS

Fall is the *Vata* season, windy and cold. Prabha Vaidya, MD, MPH, of the *Center for Holistic Medicine* explains that during this time *Vata* is the predominant energy in nature. *Vata* types may become more unbalanced and get sick. Proper precautions are necessary such as following dietary guidelines, keeping warm, and protection against wind.

Winter is *Kapha* season, when it is cold and wet. *Kapha*

types can become more unbalanced during these times. Follow a *Kapha* diet and keep warm and active.

Summer is *Pitta* season, when it is hot and dry. *Pitta* people need to avoid overheating and exercising in hot sun. Eating a *Pitta* calming diet and keeping cool will keep *Pitta* balanced.

These guidelines vary from person to person depending on their *Dosha* energies and environmental conditions.

Elaine J. Keller

Step 10:

Institute Regular Detoxes

*Detoxes are an effective way of
destroying Ama and restoring balance.*

AMA DETOX

Everyone should undergo an Ama detox at least twice a
year at the change of seasons, once at springtime, and
once again at the beginning of summer, winter or fall.

Panchakarma is a cleansing program that detoxifies the
body and mind in several stages.

The first stage involves loosening *Ama* to move it out of
tissue into the GI tract. Ingesting and applying essential
oils (oleation) get things moving, with massage and
sauna an important part of obtaining relaxation and
release. It's best to remain alone with few distractions
at this time, while engaging in meditation or prayer. A
diet of easily digestible foods like *khitchari* (see
Resources) is to be eaten during this time.

Step two is to eliminate *Ama* with the assistance of medicated enemas *(basti)* and to free up energies with nasal cleansing *(nasya)*. The *basti* process accomplishes more than simple cleansing, with herbal oil combinations eliminating toxins that have lodged deeply inside tissues. *Nasya* utilizes herb-infused oils to help you breath freely and easily.

Stage three helps to re-establish immunity and a healthy metabolism, by nourishing the body with healing practices such as yoga and meditation. *Samsarajana Karma* helps to rebuild *Agni* for proper digestion via a graduated diet. The *Remedy Guru* states that " if someone wants to kindle a large fire that can consume a large quantity of dense wood, he must begin with a spark and some blades of grass." If a log is added too quickly, it extinguishes the fire.

Thus the first meal is liquid and is taken four or five hours after the elimination stage. *Manda* is the water in which basmati rice has been boiled, and should be eaten lukewarm with a small amount of ghee and pinch of salt.

The next meal is eaten two-three hours later, and consists of eight parts water to one part rice.

The third and fourth meals consist of four parts water to one part rice. A dash of salt and a healthy sweetener such as sugar cane juice can be added, as well as ginger, turmeric, coriander, and fennel sautéed in a bit of ghee.

Cooked rice comprises the fifth meal, with yellow mung dal (Resources) as the sixth meal.

DIY PANCHAKARMA

There are many Ayurveda detox programs available online or in a retreat setting, either guided (for a cost) or unguided. These can cost upwards of several thousand dollars, and include cooking instruction and treatments as well as the detox supplies and treatments. One do-it-at home kit is compiled by Banyan Botanicals for less than $100.

Those of us unable to afford the $2500 and plus price tag for treatment at an Ayurvedic spa, have the means to implement Panchakarma at home. *NaturAsia* describes a method for do-it-yourself Panchakarma that mimics the official version quite closely. (See Resources for particulars).

Stage I – Internal Oil Application

For three consecutive days drink approx. 2oz (4 tbsp.) of warm liquid ghee on an empty stomach first thing in the morning. Vata types can add a pinch of salt to the ghee; Kapha types can add a pinch of ginger and pepper.

If you have high cholesterol, triglycerides or blood sugar levels, ghee should be substituted with flaxseed oil, 2 tablespoons, 3 times a day before meals over the course of three days.

Stage II – External Oil Application

For the next 5-7 days apply one cup of warm sesame oil over the whole body from head to foot, rubbing it in thoroughly for about 10-20 minutes. Then take a hot shower or bath, using a mild soap, allowing the protective layer of oil to remain on the skin.

Stage III – Elimination of Toxins

In the evening, approximately 1 hour after dinner, take one tablet of triphala. Alternatively take a mild laxative tea (e.g. senna), for the duration of treatment.

For the final 3 days of treatment, apply an Ayurvedic enema after a bath or shower. Enema kits can be found at any drug store or pharmacy.

When undertaking Panchakarma yourself make sure to rest as much as possible. Make yoga and meditation a part of your routine. Undergo a vegetarian diet, drink plenty of water and herbal teas , while abstaining from alcohol, coffee, tea, sweets, stimulants of any kind, and sex.

From about 5 days to the end of treatment it is advisable to eat only khitchari three times a day; with the exception of the last day of treatment when this should be eaten together with steamed vegetables. Khitchari is a nutrient-dense digestible dish favorable to all three *Doshas* for tis cleansing and balancing properties.

AFTER DETOXING

Cleansing is not enough in itself. The purification process needs to be supported by rejuvenating and restorative treatments. This maintenance prolongs the life of the cells – and thus human health and life. Panchakarma protocol calls for taking herbal pills such as ashwagandha and eating chyavanprash (Indian jam). Established supplements that nourish your body are advised as well.

Your body needs time to rejuvenate which can span a few days or several months. It is therefore necessary to continue on a healthy course of diet, exercise and meditation, says *NaturAsia*.

Elaine J. Keller

STEP-BY-STEP

THE AYURVEDA DIET GUIDELINES

STEP 1. Increase Ojas.

Nourish Yourself. Make a pre-emptive change by eliminating additives, pesticides and GMO's from your diet, and embracing foods that are wholesome. Incorporate the things that bring you harmony and joy into your lifestyle.

STEP 2. Increase Your Digestive Fire

Conduct a weekly Agni Reset until you've lost your desired amount of weight.

STEP 3. Eliminate Ama.

Eat cooked chard and kale. Steam vegetables and grains according to your Dosha. Create a detoxifying spice mixture of turmeric, coriander and fennel. Balance the six tastes, eat at the same time daily with the largest meal at noon, and never eat at night.

STEP 4. Identify Your *Dosha.*

We are each a unique combination of Vata, Pitta, and Kapha. Learn your constitutional type and areas of imbalance by taking the quizzes at the locations found in the resources.

STEP 5. Balance your *Dosha.*

Learn the six tastes and adjust your diet accordingly. Be aware of temperature and its affects, and get moving.

STEP 6. Reduce *Kapha.*

Exercise. Eliminate cold liquids and napping. Utilize herbs and avoid sweet, heavy , salty, oily, sour and greasy foods. Utilize the Mung Bean Soup Diet regularly.

STEP 7. Cook with Weight-Reducing Herbs.

Learn the spice combinations. Take Triphala and cook with fat-busting herbs.

STEP 8. Combine Your Foods.

To start with, don't eat beans with cheese. Don't eat eggs with fruit, beans, cheese, meat, or yogurt. Eat fruit alone, and never with grains.

STEP 9. Change Your Routine.

Exercise, awaken and go to sleep according to the Dosha times of the day. Be aware of, and balance seasonal effects on your Dosha.

STEP 10. Institute Regular Detoxes.

Conduct an Ama detox every spring, and at least once more in winter, summer or fall.

Elaine J. Keller

RESOURCES

DOSHA QUIZZES

Holistic Online http://www.holistic-online.com/ayurveda/ayv-diagnostic-tests.htm
Chopra Center http://DOSHAquiz.chopra.com
Ayurveda.com
http://www.ayurveda.com/pdf/constitution.pdf

RECIPES

Ghee

Heat 1lb unsalted butter in a heavy-bottomed, uncovered pan or pot
When butter is melted keep it on a steady simmer without burning (about 15 minutes).
The butter is burned if it turns brown
Blow lightly. When the liquid is transparent remove from heat.
Add a pinch of salt
Pour cooled mixture into a glass jar taking care not to include any particles, or use a fine cheesecloth or sieve. Close jar tightly. Keep covered ghee unrefrigerated as its properties improve with age. Water spoils ghee, so take care to use a dry utensil when spooning it out.

Mung Bean Soup

1 lb. green organic mung beans

4 cups water

1 tsp. turmeric

½ tsp. asafetida or hing

1 tsp. mustard seeds

2 bay leaves

Lime juice

2 Tbsp. & 2 Tbsp. chopped fresh ginger

3 cloves garlic, chopped

1 med. onion, chopped (omit for *Pitta*)

ghee

1 tsp. cumin

1 tsp. coriander powder

sea salt

Wash and soak the mung beans overnight, or at least four hours, wash and drain. Heat ghee or olive oil in a large pot and add turmeric and asafetida. Sauté for a few seconds then add the soaked beans, water and 2 Tbsp. ginger. The ratio is one part soaked mung to four parts of water. Simmer for 45 minutes, adding more water as necessary. Cook until beans are soft. In a separate pan, lightly sauté the garlic and onion in the ghee. When soft, add 2 Tbsp. finely chopped fresh root ginger. Add cumin and coriander plus remaining spices and briefly sauté. Add to mung beans and continue to simmer. Add salt to taste. Serve with a squeeze of lime and fresh coriander leaves, if desired

Detoxifying Spice Mixture (Maharishi Yoga)

1 part turmeric
2 parts ground cumin
3 parts ground coriander
4 parts ground fennel

Mix these spices together in bulk and store in a jar.
When you are cooking a meal, place a small amount of
ghee in a frying pan and heat on medium. Add
detoxifying spice mixture, measuring out one teaspoon
of spice mixture per serving of vegetables. Sauté spices
until the aroma is released (but be careful not to burn).
Add steamed vegetables, mix lightly and sauté together
for one minute. Add salt and black pepper to taste. Or
you can sauté the spice mixture in ghee and drizzle on
vegetables or grains.

Detoxifying Tea (Maharishi Yoga)

Boil two quarts of water in the morning. Add 1/4 t.
whole cumin, 1/2 t. whole coriander, 1/2 t. whole fennel
and let steep for ten minutes with the lid on. Strain out
the spices and pour water into a heat-insulating
container and sip throughout the day. Start fresh by
making a new batch of tea in the morning.

Khitchari

1 tablespoon ghee
6 ounces basmati rice
3 teaspoons cumin
 3 teaspoons coriander
3 teaspoons fennel seeds
1/2 teaspoon turmeric
3 ounces split yellow mung beans (dal)

vegetables appropriate to your *DOSHA*

Wash rice and beans together under cold water. Melt ghee in a pan and then add fennel seeds. Cook for one minute. Add cumin, coriander, and turmeric, and the rice and beans. Stir so the mixture is coated with ghee. Then cover the mixture with hot water by about two inches. Bring to a boil and then lower the heat and simmer, stirring occasionally. Add more water as needed—you don't want the pan to dry out.

Add diced vegetables, starting with root vegetables. Leafy vegetables, like spinach, should be added toward the end of cooking time. The dish is cooked when most of the water has evaporated and the grains are soft and slightly mushy.

Jau ka Pani (Barley water):

*Satisfies hunger
*Reduces cravings
*Extracts toxins from deep within the tissues
*Eliminates toxins through the urinary tract
*Is diuretic
*Relieves fluid retention
*Balance Kapha
*Helps metabolize and eliminate fat
*Promotes weight loss

Drink 6 cups of Barley water every day and keep regular exercise regime.

Note: Do not drink after 6pm to avoid disturbing sleep due to the diuretic effect.

Boil one handful of whole grain (not "pealed") barley in 6 cups of water for 15 minutes. Strain the barley out and pour the water into a thermos. Drink the water throughout the day.

SOURCES FOR RAW HONEY, RAW MILK, RAW BUTTER (FOR GHEE) AND NON-GMO ORGANIC FOOD:

Please note: there are no kick-backs from or affiliations with any company mentioned. We do not receive a percentage if you follow these links.

Green Polka Dot Box
www.Greenpolkadotbox.com

Living Honey
www.livinghoney.biz

Real Milk Finder
http://www.realmilk.com/real-milk-finder/

Really Raw Honey
https://sites.google.com/site/spiritualfoodcsa/food-a-pedia/raw-honey

Some info on Ayurveda and honey:
http://sanyoga-ayurveda.blogspot.com/2010/11/why-honey-and-ghee-mixed-is-poison.html

AMA DETOX SHOPPING LIST AND INSTRUCTIONS

100% Pure Sesame Oil

Hobe Naturals
http://www.hobelabs.com

Saquuin (on *Amazon*)
http://www.*Amazon*.com/Sesame-Seed-Oil-Refined-100/dp/B005791TTU

Banyan Botanicals (32 oz.)
http://www.banyanbotanicals.com/prodinfo.asp?number=3141

Triphala and Senna (see Herb Sources)

DIY Ayurvedic Enema or Basti Instructions

Yogi Times
http://www.yogitimes.com/article/enema-ayurveda-cleaning-colon-hydrotherapy-colonic-natural/

Shaktiveda on YouTube
http://www.youtube.com/watch?v=wvBB3ZqJDPE

Ayurvedic Institute
http://www.ayurveda.com/pdf/basti_colon_cleansing.pdf

Enema Bag (any drugstore)

KAPALABHATI INSTRUCTIONS

http://www.abc-of-yoga.com/pranay*Ama*/basic/kapal.asp

GUIDED PANCHAKARMA

Retreat Finder
http://www.skinnydivadiet.com/2012/09/spas-and-centers-offering-panchakarma.html

FOOD TASTE LISTS

BITTER *lessens Kapha and Pitta, increases Vata*

Brussels sprouts
Chicory
Citrus peel
Cloves
Cocoa
Coffee
Dark chocolate
Dill
Eggplant
Fenugreek
Grapefruit
Green cabbage
Kale
Mustard greens
Olives (uncured)
Radicchio
Spinach
Spinach
Zucchini/courgette

PUNGENT *lessens Kapha, increases Pitta and Vata*

Anchovies
Anise
Black pepper
Brie cheese
Cardamom
Cauliflower
Chili
Cinnamon
Cloves
Cumin
Garlic
Ginger
Horseradish
Kimchee
Mint
Mustard
Mustard seeds
Onion
Oregano
Radish
Red pepper
Sardines
Thyme
Turmeric

ASTRINGENT *lessens Kapha and Pitta, increases Vata*

Apples
Artichoke
Asparagus
Beans
Berries
Broccoli
Buckwheat
Cauliflower

Cranberries
Hazelnuts
Honey
Jasmine
Lentils
Most raw vegetables
Pears
Peas
Persimmon
Pomegranate
Quinoa
Rye
Sprouts
Turmeric
Walnuts

SALTY *lessens Vata, increases Kapha and Pitta*

Any kind of salt such as rock salt, sea salt, and salt from
the ground; any food to which salt has been added

SOUR *lessens Vata, increases Kapha and Pitta*

Lemon
Lime
passion fruit
sour cherries
plum
tamarind
yogurt
cheese
whey
sour cream
fermented substances such as wine, vinegar, soy sauce,
or sour cabbage; carbonated beverages (including soft
drinks or beer)

SWEET *lessens Pitta and Vata, increases Kapha*

Wheat
Rice
Barley
Corn
Ghee
Cream
butter
dates
figs
grapes
pear
coconut
mango
potato
carrot
cauliflower
string beans
sugar in any form such as raw, refines, brown, white, molasses, and sugar cane juice

AYURVEDIC HERB SOURCES

Ayurveda for You http://ayurveda-foryou.com
Ayurveda Herbs http://www.ayurveda-herbs.com
Banyan Botanicals http://www.banyanbotanicals.com
Gopalan Organics http://www.gopalanorganics.com/
Jade Dragon Online http://www.jadedragon.com
Lotus Blooming Herbs
http://www.authenticshilajit.com/
Maharisha Ayurveda
http://mapi.com/maharishi_ayurveda
Native Remedies http://www.nativeremedies.com
Pukka Incredible Organic Herbs
http://www.pukkaherbs.com

REFERENCES

Soni Yoga
http://soniyoga.com

The Secrets of Ayurveda, Vaidya Suresh Chaturvedi
http://pustak.org

Eat, Taste, Heal, An Ayurvedic Cookbook for Modern
Living
http://www.eattasteheal.com

Ayurveda *DOSHA*
http://ayurveda*DOSHA*.org

Mind, Body, Green
http://www.mindbodygreen.com

Yoga Journal
http://www.yogajournal.com

Ayurveda Info center at Holistic Online
http://www.holistic-online.com

Banyan Botanicals
http://www.banyanbotanicals.com

Traditional Indian Herb directory

http://mobsea.co/hm/

Ayurveda for you
http://ayurveda-foryou.com

Physiological aspects of Agni
http://www.ncbi.nlm.nih.gov/pmc/articles/PMC32210
79/

The Chopra Center
http://www.chopra.com

Yachna Yoga
http://yachnayoga.wordpress.com/yoga-asans

Ill Wind BlogSpot
http://illwindblog.blogspot.com/2010/02/*Agni*-and-
Ama-ayurvedic-perspective-on.html

Taranco Wellness Center
http://tarancowellness.com

Med India Net
http://www.medindia.net/patients/lifestyleandwellnes
s/herbs-for-weight-loss-pros-and-cons-
supplements.htm

Ayurvedic Treatment Guide
http://www.ayurveda-treatment-guide.com

Mother Earth Living
http://www.motherearthliving.com/health-and-
wellness

A Beginner's Guide to Ayurveda
http://heymonicab.com/ayurveda-an-overview

Ayurvedic Florida
http://ayurveda-florida.com/

DOSHA Balance
http://www.DOSHAbalance.com

The Living Centre
http://www.thelivingcentre.com

The Ayurveda Way
http://q-theayurvedaway.blogspot.com.au

Ayurveda Alchemy
http://www.ayurvedaalchemy.com/

Holistic Medicine
http://www.centerforholisticmedicine.com/

Chepulis, L M. The effect of honey compared to sucrose, mixed sugars, and a sugar-free diet on weight gain in young rats. Journal of Food Science, 2007; 72; 3: S224-S229.

Sebastian Pole
http://www.sanatansociety.org

Elaine J. Keller

THE FOLLOWING PAGES
ARE FORMATTED FOR YOU TO
CUT OUT OR PHOTOCOPY.
HANG THEM IN YOUR KITCHEN
OR CARRY THEM WITH YOU FOR
REFERENCE

Elaine J. Keller

TO CREATE OJAS

Practice yoga & *Prana Ama* breathing exercises
Get plenty of physical activity
Be positive!
Balance your diet with the six food tastes
Laugh often!
Follow your path in life. Give to others. Learn to receive.
Nourish yourself
Enjoy orgasms with the correct partner
Work on your digestion
Eat sweet foods like dates, seeds and nuts like almonds
Eat *Chyavanprash* (Ayurvedic jam)
Eat around people you enjoy
Meditate
Practice *Bhakti* yoga (devotion)
Learn controlled release of sexual energy
Cook with *Ghee*

Elaine J. Keller

AGNI RESET

DAY 1
Normal breakfast and lunch. Light, nourishing dinner.
Before bed: 3 tablets *senna*, followed by a glass of hot water.
Go to bed early.

DAY 2
Only drinks. Organic Apple or grape juice heated by adding
hot water. One glass at breakfast, one at lunch one at dinner.
Drink only three more during the day, otherwise drink water.
Be aware that toxins going into the mind are as harmful as
physicals toxins.

DAY 3
Light breakfast of hot cereal with a cup of licorice tea for
*Vata*s, peppermint tea for *Pitta*s and *Kapha*s. Have a second
helping of cereal if you need it. Do not eat again until noon
when you should cook up a substantial, nourishing lunch.
Drink ginger tea .
Light dinner at least three hours before bed.

RESET RULES
Avoid alcohol, caffeine and cigarettes
Eat at regular times and don't snack between meals
Keep salt to a minimum and only have it with food
Stick to recipes with foods appropriate to your *DOSHA*
If you get faint on Day 2, add honey to your warm juice
Don't skip meals, unless you are *Kapha*

INCREASING *AGNI*
Cook with ginger, cayenne, and other warming spices
Drink a warm cup of ginger tea before meals, or suck on a
piece of raw ginger sprinkled with lemon juice to fire
digestion.

Elaine J. Keller

FOOD TASTE LISTS

BITTER *lessens Kapha and Pitta, increases Vata*

Brussels sprouts
Chicory
Citrus peel
Cloves
Cocoa
Coffee
Dark chocolate
Dill
Eggplant
Fenugreek
Grapefruit
Green cabbage
Kale
Mustard greens
Olives (uncured)
Radicchio
Spinach
Spinach
Zucchini/courgette

PUNGENT *lessens Kapha, increases Pitta and Vata*

Anchovies
Anise
Black pepper
Brie cheese
Cardamom
Cauliflower
Chili
Cinnamon
Cloves
Cumin
Garlic
Ginger
Horseradish
Kimchee
Mint
Mustard
Mustard seeds
Onion
Oregano
Radish
Red pepper
Sardines
Thyme
Turmeric

ASTRINGENT *lessens Kapha and Pitta, increases Vata*

Apples
Artichoke
Asparagus
Beans
Berries
Broccoli
Buckwheat
Cauliflower
Cranberries
Hazelnuts
Honey
Jasmine
Lentils
Most raw vegetables
Pears
Peas
Persimmon
Pomegranate
Quinoa
Rye
Sprouts
Turmeric
Walnuts

SALTY *lessens Vata, increases Kapha and Pitta*

Any kind of salt or salted food

SOUR *lessens Vata, increases Kapha and Pitta*

Lemon
Lime
passion fruit
sour cherries
plum
tamarind
yogurt
cheese

whey
sour cream
fermented substances such as
wine, vinegar, soy sauce, or
sour cabbage; carbonated
beverages (including soft
drinks or beer)

SWEET
lessens Pitta and Vata, increases Kapha

Wheat
Rice
Barley
Corn
Ghee
Cream
butter
dates
figs
grapes
pear

coconut
mango
potato
carrot
cauliflower
string beans
sugar in any form such as
raw, refines, brown, white,
molasses, and sugar cane
juice

Elaine J. Keller

TO ELIMINATE AMA, AID DIGESTION & REDUCE WEIGHT

Cook With :

Aloe Vera
Asafetida (*hing*)
Ashwagandha
Barberry
Black pepper
Cardamom
Cayenne pepper
Celery seed, leaf, root, stalk
Chitrak
Cinnamon
Coriander
Cumin
Fennel, Fennel seeds

Fresh curry leaves
Ginger root
Guduchi
Guggulu (take with Triphala)
Gymnema sylvestre
Kalijeera (bitter cumin)
Mustard seed
Neem
Pippali (if *ama* is in excess*)
Trikatu
Triphala
Turmeric

Utilize:

Chyawanprash
Kitchari
Castor oil in small quantities
Emphasize bitter, mildly spicy and astringent flavors.
Cooked leafy greens such as chard and kale
Steamed vegetables and grains with spices suitable for your type
Churna
Shilajit

Avoid (*especially during detoxification periods*):

cold drinks, carbonated drinks, alcohol, caffeine, dairy products,
tobacco, sweet fruit , sweetened food, wheat, pastries, bread,
meat, fish, and eggs

Elaine J. Keller

EASILY DIGESTED FOODS

Grains: Aged rice, millet, wheat, oats, couscous, rye, barley, amaranth

Cooked Vegetables: Squash, okra, radish, eggplant, sweet potato, bamboo shoots, bitter melon, spinach, onion, daikon radish, avocado, carrots, broccoli, parsnip, beets, asparagus, artichoke, bok choy, brussel spouts, burdock root, cabbage, cauliflower, green beans, leafy greens, peas, turnips, cauliflower, zucchini, kohlarabi, leeks

Fruits*:* Coconut, grapes, mango, apricot, raisins, strawberries, pomegranates, persimmons, cranberries, banana, berries, cherries, figs, dates, grapefruit, kiwi, lemons, limes, oranges, papaya, plums, rhubarb, prunes, pears

Legumes *(soaked and well cooked):*Mung beans, aduki beans, red lentils, chana dal, black-eyed peas, garbanzo, kidney beans, black beans, split peas, white beans, navy beans, pinto beans

Nuts & Seeds*:* Sesame seeds, almonds, charoli, pumpkin seeds, brazil nuts, cashews, coconut, hazelnut, macadamia nut, pecans, pistachio, walnuts, chia, flax seeds, sunflower seeds, hemp seeds, poppy seeds

Fresh Dairy*:* Raw cow's milk, ghee, butter, goat milk, home made buttermilk, unsalted cheese

Meat*:* Buffalo, bone broth, goat, rabbit, chicken, turkey, lamb

Occasional: beef, fish, seafood, duck, chicken eggs, duck eggs, pig

Sweeteners*:* Raw honey, jaggery, rock sugar, raw sugar cane, 100% pure maple syrup, sucanat, agave, turbinado sugar

Oils: Sesame, ghee, unsalted butter, olive oil, peanut oil, coconut oil, flax oil (never heat), hemp oil, pumpkin seed oil

FOOD COMBINATIONS

Don't combine:

Beans *with...*	... fruit, cheese, eggs, fish, milk, meat, yogurt
Eggs *with...*	...fruit, especially melons, beans, cheese, fish, khitchari, MILK (especially), meat, yogurt
Fruit *with...*	... any other food.
Grains *with...*	...fruit (esp. acidic or sour taste), tapioca
Honey *with...*	... ghee
Hot drinks *with...*	... mangos, cheese, fish, meat, starch, yogurt
Lemon *with...*	... cucumbers, milk, tomatoes, yogurt
Melons *with...*	...eat alone.
Milk *with...*	... BANANAS (especially), cherries, melons, sour fruits; bread containing yeast, fish, khitchari, meat, yogurt
Nightshades *with...* (i.e. potato, tomato)	... melon, cucumber, dairy products
Radishes *with...*	... bananas, raisins; milk
Tapioca *with...*	... fruit, especially banana and mango; beans, raisins, jaggery
Yogurt *with...*	... fruit, cheese, eggs, fish, hot drinks, meat
Milk *with...*	Milk with... nightshades

Elaine J. Keller

www.ingramcontent.com/pod-product-compliance
Lightning Source LLC
Chambersburg PA
CBHW060510280326
41933CB00014B/2908